Fifty Years of Clinical Holistic Treatment for Parkinson's

· A UNIQUE APPROACH ·

SEIYU KAGEYAMA

Fifty Years of Clinical Holistic Treatment for Parkinson's
A Unique Approach

iUniverse books may be ordered through booksellers or by contacting:

iUniverse
1663 Liberty Drive
Bloomington, IN 47403
www.iuniverse.com
1-800-Authors (1-800-288-4677)

ISBN: 978-1-5320-8040-1 (sc)
ISBN: 978-1-5320-8041-8 (e)

Library of Congress Control Number: 2019913010

Print information available on the last page.

iUniverse rev. date: 10/23/2019

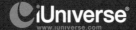

FIFTY YEARS OF CLINICAL HOLISTIC TREATMENT FOR PARKINSON'S

A **Unique** Approach

Contents

ABOUT THE AUTHOR

Seiyu Kageyama was born in China and is a naturalized citizen of Japan. He has been assiduously trained in internal strength and martial arts and diligently learned Chinese acupuncture from his father, taking a hands-on approach. He has nearly fifty years of experience in clinical treatment.

One of the most memorable days was when his father taught him how to use Mang Zhen (芒针), the special needle that is more than seventy centimeters long. Mang Zhen is used to puncture the Dai Mai (带脉) channel, crossing through inner organs in the abdomen on one side to reach the Dai Mai on the other side of the body. It was said throughout the three thousand years of acupuncture history in China, only two or three people have practiced this technology.

In the decades following clinical practice, Mr. Kageyama continued to research and explore the treatment of Parkinson's disease, finally discovering his method in 2007. In the twelve years leading up to the publication of this book, experience has shown that if patients are continuously treated, this method can restore their lives to normal.

Through Mr. Kageyama's unique and special treatment, not only can Parkinson's patients recover but so can those suffering from other kinds of diseases such as hypertension, rheumatoid arthritis, climacteric syndrome, postpartum depression, cervical spondylosis, acid reflux, allergies, and eczema. Furthermore, Mr. Kageyama can help people consistently to regain fresh blood to obtain beautiful skin and an energetic appearance, along with feeling younger and living longer.

If you are interested, you can get a lot of inspiration from the ancient Chinese classical medical books represented by Huangdi Neijing from three thousand years ago.

Licenses
National acupuncturist license of Japan
Acupuncturist license, California, United States

Awards and Acknowledgments

2007: the first rehabilitated Parkinson's disease in Japan

2010: Parkinson's Therapy Excellent Paper Award, WFAS 2010 International Acupuncture Conference in the United States, presidium of the general assembly

2015: performance of treating Parkinson's patients at the VA treatment center in San Francisco, which worked immediately and was called a "miracle"

2016: Parkinson Patient Conference with a thousand people in attendance, Hollywood star Michael J. Fox Foundation, World Parkinson Conference with 4,500 people (Portland, Oregon)

2019: Japan Kyoto World Parkinson Conference with nearly ten thousand patients, American Parkinson Disease Association USA

Medical Revolution Knowledge and Mythology on Parkinson Rehabilitation Special Treatment

Chinese Ancestral Acupuncture, Kung Fu Acupoint Manipulation, Meridian and Collaterals Cell Recovery Technology

1 Introduction

The British doctor James Parkinson named this disease after himself in 1817. It has been used for two hundred years since then. The world's advanced research, led by the United States, has involved hundreds of billions of dollars and tens of thousands of scientific experts researching Parkinson's treatment. However, experts are still struggling and concentrating on Western medicine and mythology.

From a Chinese medicine point of view, everyone has a self-healing functionality to restore body health, particularly functional disease. Chinese medicine has the best recovery treatment from restoration. Parkinson's disease is a typical syndrome that begins to develop from the midbrain and affects every organ in the brain and body to make its functionality chaotic until patients pass away.

As of now, the etiology, pathology, diagnosis, and symptoms of Parkinson's syndrome have been recognized as the following, and my explanation may look repetitious as reported from others, but I can show you more detail along with my illustrations.

1.1 Disease Cause

Most of the cause of Parkinson's disease is unknown. A small related possibility can be from genetic factors. Some other risk factors may also be associated with Parkinson's disease, but the cause-and-effect correlation has not been approved.

1.2 Genetic Factor

Traditionally thought, Parkinson's disease is not a hereditary disease. In fact, 15 percent of Parkinson's patients in first-degree family relatives (including parents, children, and siblings) have the same problem. It is known that at least 5 percent of Parkinson's disease is caused by mutations in one or several specific genes.

It has been confirmed that specific gene mutations cause Parkinson's disease. The proteins encoded by these genes include α-Synuclein (SNCA), Parkin (PRKN), PARK8 (LRRK2, also known as tremor), PTEN-induced kinase, (PINK1), DJ-1, and ATP13A2.

Except for LRRK2, patients with these mutations usually suffer from Parkinson's disease. Dual LRRK2 mutations cause only a small amount of people to get sick. SNCA and LRRK2 encompass the most advanced research on Parkinson's disease–related genes. SNCA, LRRK2, and glucocerebrosidase (GBA) mutations increase the risk of sporadic Parkinson's disease and cause Gaucher's disease. Researchers have used genome-wide association analysis to search for mutant alleles with low penetrance in sporadic Parkinson's disease and collected many positive results.

Since α-Synuclein is a component of Lewy's, the SNCA gene is extremely important for Parkinson's disease. The SNCA gene in a familial Parkinson's disease may have missense mutations (a changed single nucleotide causing amino acid distortion) and replicate two or three times. The missense mutations are rare, but genetic duplication causes about 2 percent of families with Parkinson's disease. Some people with Parkinson's disease can also find mutations in the SNCA gene, but they are not diagnosed because of insufficient penetrance or the potential patients in young age.

The protein encoded by the LRRK2 gene is also named tremor. Since the gene was originally discovered in the families of England and Northern Spain, its name *dardarin* in English is derived from the "trembling" of the Basque language. Mutations in the LRRK2 gene are the most commonly known causes of incidental Parkinson's disease, which encompasses about 5 percent of patients with a family history and 3 percent of sporadic patients. There are so many types of mutations, but only a few types have confirmed the cause of this disease.

Partial Parkinson's disease is related to genes and digestive functions of the solution. So there are studies speculating that Parkinson's disease may be related to the malfunction of the solution, which will cause the cells to be unable to break down α-Synuclein.

1.3 Anatomy

The main pathological distortion in Parkinson's disease occurs in the ventral part of the cerebral substantia nigra. This area contains many dopamine neurons and acts as a transmitter to the basal ganglia of the brain. In patients with this disease, many neurons that are densified around the body are malfunctioning or blocked. Some even lose up to 70 percent of the neurons.

Usually a normal person's blue nucleus and substantia nigra are darker colored because cells in this area produce neuromelanin. In the case of Parkinson's disease, the blue nucleus and nigra are lighter because of the massive death of neurons. Under microscopic observation, it is noticed that the number of neurons in the substantia nigra are reduced and the Lewy bodies are in the remnants of the cells.

At the same time, the stellate cells will die along with the neurons, and the microglia cells will activate to clear the cell debris. Among them, Lewy bodies in Parkinson's disease have the most distinguishing pathological features.

1.4 Pathophysiology

The main symptoms of Parkinson's disease are mostly due to the degradation of dopaminergic neurons in the substantia nigra pars compacta.

The path connecting the basal ganglia of the brain to the outside world can be divided into five sectors according to its projection position: action circuit, ocular eye circuit, combined cortical circuit, edge system circuit, and orbital frontal skin circuit. Because Parkinson's disease affects the transmission of information upstream of the basal ganglia, all the circuits are affected. Then the Parkinson's patient has movement, attention, and learning obstacles. Up to now, the best thorough research is the impact of the disease on the motor circuit.

In 1980, the theoretical prototype of the motor circuit and the association of the circuit with Parkinson's disease were brought to the attention of the scientific community at that time. Later it was discovered that the model could not explain certain phenomena, and the corrections were made.

In this model, the basal ganglia are responsible for in-progress motion systems to avoid inappropriate timing activation. When the brain determines certain movement is to be performed, the basal ganglia will reduce the signal of suppression so the action can be performed smoothly. Dopamine can inhibit the inhibition information from the basal ganglia. Therefore, high-density dopamine can promote the smooth occurrence of motion commands, and when the dopamine concentration is low, the motion command will receive the inhibition from the basal ganglia.

Parkinson's patients have lower concentrations of central nervous system dopamine, resulting in decreased motor function. Based on this theory, medications that increase the concentration of dopamine are often used in drug therapy, but the result also leads to the activation of the motor system at an inappropriate time, causing involuntary body movements.

1.5 Brain Neuron Death

The cause of Parkinson's disease creating dopamine neuron death is still undecided. It is theoretically believed that because the patient's α-Synuclein accumulates and binds to ubiquitin, it results in cell destruction. These poorly soluble proteins are deposited in the cell body to form Lewy bodies.

According to the Braque analyzation, Lewy bodies first appear in the olfactory bulb, medulla, and pons. The patients at this stage had no obvious symptoms. As the disease progresses, Lewy bodies appear in the substantia nigra and the base of the forebrain. And finally they appear in the neocortex, which is also the brain area where the patient is mainly injured.

However, it is also believed that Lewy bodies do not necessarily lead to cell death and may even be a protective protein. The cerebral cortex of dementia patients is also common in Lewy bodies, but the characteristics of Alzheimer's disease, such as nerve fiber entanglement and age spots, are only present in patients with dementia.

Proteasome disability, loss of function, and decreased mitochondrial activity are also mechanisms of cell death. Ion accumulation in the substantia nigra cells is often accompanied by protein inclusions, which may be related to oxidative stress, protein sets, and neuronal cell death, but the exact mechanism remains unclear.

1.6 Diagnosis

In the diagnosis of Parkinson's disease and the history of neurological examination, there is no experimental test method that can effectively prove Parkinson's disease, but brain imaging can sometimes rule out other diseases with similar symptoms. The improvement in motor symptoms after taking L-dopa can help the doctor confirm that the patient is suffering from Parkinson's disease.

If you can find Lewy bodies in the midbrain during an autopsy, it means that the patient had suffered from Parkinson's disease in his lifetime. As the disease progresses, there are naturally occurring symptoms of Parkinson's disease, and the doctor might accidentally rule out the possibility of Parkinson's disease. Therefore, some authoritative guidelines recommend that doctors must regularly review the diagnosis of Parkinson's disease patients.

Other diseases may indirectly cause Parkinson's, including Alzheimer's disease, multiple cerebral infarction, and drug induction. Differential diagnosis must exclude Parkinson's additional syndrome (such as progressive upper nucleus and multiple systemic degeneration). Anti-Parkinson's drugs are usually ineffective for Parkinson's additional syndrome.

If the patient's symptoms worsen quicker, for instance, early cognitive difficulties, unstable posture, mild tremors, or both sides of body, it means that he is suffering from Parkinson's additional syndrome instead of simple Parkinson's disease. Hereditary Parkinson's syndrome is usually classified as Parkinson's disease. Also, the familial Parkinson's disease and the familial Parkinson's additional syndrome are used to express as the same disease.

Medical institutions have established a guideline for diagnostic conditions for Parkinson's disease to simplify and standardize this process, which is especially useful in the early stages of the disease. The most widely known of these are the Brain Bank of the Parkinson's Association of the United Kingdom and the National Center for Neurological Disorders and Stroke.

The Brain Bank defines the slowness of motion as a diagnostic requirement for Parkinson's disease, and at the same time, the patient has at least one of the symptoms of limb stiffness, restless tremor, or stance. The possibility of other diseases must be excluded.

As the disease progresses, the patient symptoms must also have the following characteristics: unilateral seizures, restless tremors, disease progression over time, asymmetry of motor symptoms, response to L-dopa therapy for more than five years, clinical course more than ten years, overdose of L-dopa causing difficulty in sports, and so on. According to the evaluation of pathological anatomy, the accuracy of the above diagnostic conditions is about 75 to 90 percent, and the diagnosis made by experts, such as neurologists, has a higher accuracy.

Computed tomography (CT) and magnetic resonance imaging (MRI) in the brain of patients with Parkinson's disease appear to be the same as normal, but these techniques can be used to rule out other indirect causes of Parkinson's syndrome, such as basal ganglia tumors, vascular lesions, and cerebral edema. It has been reported that diffusion MRI helps distinguish between typical and atypical Parkinson's syndrome, but its exact diagnostic power is still under investigation.

The dopamine function of the basal ganglia can be measured by radiography techniques such as positron emission computed tomography (PET) and single photon emission computed tomography (SPECT), such as iodine-Flupan (Io-123) used in SPECT (trade name DaTSCAN) and iodotropen (Dopascan), as well as fluorodeoxyglucose and DTBZ used in PET. Decreased dopamine activity in the basal ganglia can also aid in the diagnosis of Parkinson's disease.

1.7 Neuropathic Disorder

Parkinson's disease can be from mild to severe neuropsychiatric disorders, including speech, cognition, mood, behavior, and confusion. There may be cognitive confusion in the early stages of the disease and sometimes even before the diagnosis of Parkinson's disease. The prevalence rate correlates to the duration of illness. The most common cognitive deficit in patients with Parkinson's disease is implementation difficulties, which will affect patients' planning, cognitive flexibility, abstract thinking, regulation understanding, appropriate behavior, memorization, concentration, all aspects, and so forth.

Cognitive difficulties also include distraction of attention, inaccurate time perception and estimation, and deceleration of cognitive processing. The patient's memory is affected. It is especially difficult to recall the previous learning knowledge; however, providing clues to assist the patient's recall can improve the associated symptoms. Losing the sense of space is another possible symptom. During diagnosis, the patient is asked to identify the facial expression and the direction of the line to determine whether the patient has such an obstacle.

The risk of Parkinson's disease is 2.6 times higher than the average person, and the incidence increases as the duration of illness. Dementia and caregiver might live in lower quality of life, higher rate in mortality, and higher possibility to live in a nursing home.

Compared with the average person, patients with Parkinson's disease without cognitive impairment are most likely to have behavioral and emotional disorders and not to have dementia. The most common mood disorders are depression, apathy, and anxiety. However, a Parkinson's patient often has symptoms such as dementia, fewer facial expressions, diminishing motor function, apathy, and difficulty in making vocalization. All above make emotional-disorder diagnoses much more complicated.

Patients with Parkinson's disease may also have issues with drug abuse and addiction, ecstasy, hypersexuality, gambling, or impulsive behavior control. Those may be related to the medication during treatment. About 4 percent of Parkinson's patients suffer from symptoms of hallucinations or delusions. These psychiatric symptoms are generally the result of excessive dopamine during treatment, so the longer the disease or the more L-dopa patients have taken, it also easier runs into these symptoms.

1.8 Other Symptoms

Sleep disorders are also a possible symptom of Parkinson's disease, and treatments may worsen the problem. Patients with sleepiness, interruption of REM, insomnia, and so on, according to a systematic review, showed that 13 percent of patients with Parkinson's disease taking dopamine caused sleep problems.

Changes in the autonomic nervous system may introduce postural hypotension, oily skin, excessive sweating, urinary incontinence, and sexual dysfunction. Patients may also experience severe constipation and abnormal gastrointestinal motility, causing extreme discomfort and harmed health.

Parkinson's disease is also associated with some eye diseases and visual abnormalities, including reduction in blinking frequency, dry eye, chasing disorder, saccade (both eyes beating in the same direction by autonomic nerves), inability to stare upward, blurred vision, and diplopia. Sensory problems may be manifested in loss of smell or pain and paresthesia (stinging and numbness of the skin). All the above autonomic and sensory symptoms happen one year before the patient's diagnosis.

1.9 Social Expenditure

Parkinson's disease presents a huge social burden. The actual amount is difficult to calculate due to methodological and countrywide issues. The amount of Parkinson's disease in the United Kingdom is estimated to be between £3.3 and 4.49 billion per year. In the United States, it is about $230 billion dollars, and the average annual cost per patient is about $10,000. The largest cost is for hospitalization and care. Next is the cost of medicine.

According to statistics from Shanghai, China, in 2006, each person with Parkinson's disease spends an average of 7,679 RMB per year, which is half of the local average income. The largest expense comes from drug costs. In addition to the main costs, Parkinson's disease also brings huge indirect costs, such as the decline in patient productivity and the labor and financial burden of caregiver at home. It affects the quality of life of both parties.

1.10 Initiative Promotion

To raise public awareness of the disease, the European Parkinson's Association has named James Parkinson's birthday (April 11) as the annual World Parkinson's Day. In 2005, international organizations selected red tulips as a symbol of the disease because the Dutch horticulturist JWS Van der Wereld named the cultivar he cultivated in 1981 as "James Parkinson Tulips."

The Parkinson Foundation of the United States has provided $180 million annually from 1982 to sponsor Parkinson's care, research, and services. William Black founded the Parkinson's Disease Foundation in 1957. Since its inception, he has donated $115 million in research and $50 million in education and outreach programs. Others include the American Parkinson's Association, founded in 1961, and the European Parkinson's Association, established in 1992.

1.11 Famous Examples

Actor Michael J. Fox brought public attention to the disease after being diagnosed with Parkinson's disease. After the diagnosis, Fox chose to face the disease, even without taking the medicine and still performing on public programs, letting people realize the impact of the disease. He also wrote two autobiographies describing his journey against the disease. In addition, Fox has also explained the impact of the disease to the US Congress without taking medicine and established the Michael J. Fox Foundation to find a way to cure Parkinson's disease. Caroline College awarded him a honorary medical doctorate for his support and contribution to research on Parkinson's disease.

At the age of forty, the Olympic bronze medalist Davis Finney discovered he had Parkinson's disease. Finney founded the Davis Finney Foundation in 2004 to fund research related to improving patients' quality of life.

Mohammad Ali had symptoms of Parkinson's disease at the age of thirty-eight but was not diagnosed until he was forty-two years old. He was known as the world's best-known patient with Parkinson's disease. But Ali was suffering from Parkinson's disease or boxer-type dementia. So far, there is still no clue.

Former Chinese leader Deng Xiaoping also suffered from Parkinson's disease. He had been suffering from dyspnea, swallowing disorders, coughing, and other symptoms for more than ten years. He also needed machine-assisted breathing and died on February 19, 1997, because of respiratory failure.

2 Motor Symptoms

2.1 Symptoms

Parkinson's disease has motor and nonmotor symptoms, including autonomic nervous system dysfunction, neuropsychiatric disorders (including emotion, cognition, behavior, and mind changes), sensation, and sleep disorders. Some nonmotor symptoms often appear at the time of diagnosis and may even occur earlier than exercise symptoms.

2.2 Motor Symptoms

There are seven main motor symptoms in Parkinson's disease: trembling, limb stiffness, deceleration in movement, unstable posture and short steps, facial features unable to show laughter, stiff tongue and unclear speech, and written words gradually become smaller.

Trembling is the most obvious and best-known symptom. About 30 percent of patients with Parkinson's disease do not tremble at the beginning stage, but as time passes, most patients will gradually develop this symptom. The tremor of Parkinson's disease is usually a static tremor. That is, the limbs are most stunned when they are at rest, but the symptoms disappear when sleeping or consciously moving the limbs.

Trembling symptoms will have an extreme impact on the future of disease development. Usually the symptom happens in one hand or one foot at the time of onset but then spreads to both hands and feet. The tremor frequency of Parkinson's disease is between 4 and 6 Hertz, often accompanied with the hand movement of "making small dough." That is, the patient's index finger will involuntarily move closer to the thumb so the two fingers circle each other as if the pharmacist is making pills.

Hypokinesia is another hallmark of Parkinson's disease. The patient's movements slow down and affect the entire process from the beginning of the exercise to the execution. The patient cannot make continuous actions or perform different actions simultaneously. Bradykinesia is a type of hypokinesia that is slow movements during exercise and is a common symptom at an early stage of Parkinson's disease.

Patients initially encounter difficulties in performing daily activities such as writing, sewing, or dressing. Clinical evaluators observe patients while performing the above actions. The effects of bradykinesia are varied with the type of action and mental state of the patient. The patient's activity and emotional state affect the degree of influence. Some patients are no longer able to walk, but others are still able to ride a bicycle. In general, patients with Parkinson's disease can improve the symptoms of bradykinesia after treatment.

Rigidity is due to an increase in muscle tone and a constant muscle contraction, which makes limbs difficult to move. Limb stiffness caused by Parkinson's may be lead-tube stiffness (fixed resistance) or gear stiffness (resistance not fitness but regular), and increased tremor and muscle tone may cause gear stiffness. Limb stiffness may also be associated with joint pain, which is often seen in the patient's early stages. The limb stiffness of Parkinson's early patients often happens in the arms and occurs around the neck and shoulders. It then spreads to the face and limbs. Finally it spreads to the whole body as the disease progresses, causing the patient to gradually lose exercise capacity.

Postural instability is a typical symptom of Parkinson's disease last stage. Patients often fall due to a loss of balance and often suffer from fractures. In the early stages of the disease, there is usually a stint of instability, especially for the elderly. Up to 40 percent of patients have fallen due to unstable posture, and 10 percent of patients have fallen at least once a week. The number of falls is related to the severity of the illness.

Other motor signs of Parkinson's disease also include posture, speech, and swallowing abnormalities. Patients may have flurried gait (accelerated when walking and staggering) to avoid falling. They may also experience difficulties or masklike faces, or their written words get smaller and smaller, along with various sports problems.

3 Twelve O'Clock Sectors and Human Body Meridian Timetable

Next, let's look at the relationship between the body's meridian direction and the body structure relation.

3.1 Chou

The time of liver detoxification operation is 1:00 a.m. to 3:00 a.m. (Chou). The liver is prosperous. At Chou, if you do not sleep late, then your face won't grow pigments. According to the traditional Chinese medicine theory, "the liver is holding blood" and "when the person is lying, the blood flows to the liver."

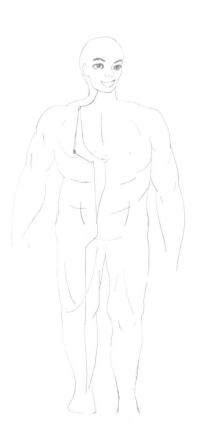

If the person can't fall asleep during Chou, the liver is still outputting energy to support a person's thinking and actions, and the metabolism cannot be completed. Therefore, for the person who failed to fall asleep before the Chou time, his face turns a green and gray color. His emotions are decelerating and embarrassing. He is prone to liver disease, and his face is dark and grows pigments.

Deficiency Syndrome
Fatigue, loss of vision, decreased sexual function, dizziness, yellow skin, and so on

Empirical Syndrome
Irascibility flourishing, tempered, dizziness, low back pain, menstrual disorders, insomnia, and intercostal neuralgia

3.2 Yin

The time when the lungs run through the hole is 3:00 a.m. to 5:00 a.m. (Yin). In Yin, the lungs are prosperous if the sleep is deep, and then the face is rosy and full of energy.

"The lungs have a hundred veins."

After the liver blows the blood out of the Chou, the blood is supplied to the lungs and sent to the whole body through the lungs. Therefore, people look rosy and energetic in the morning. In Yin, people with lung disease have the strongest symptoms, such as terrible cough or asthma. They are woken up from the suffering of sickness.

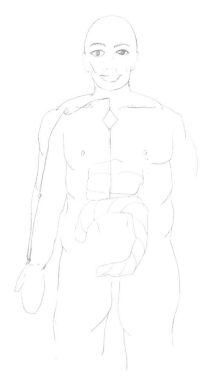

Deficiency Syndrome
Reduced skin immunity, cold hands and feet, paralysis, dry throat, cough, and so on

Empirical Syndrome
Difficulty breathing, throat problems, chest tightness, asthma, tonsillitis, cough, shoulder pain, susceptibility to hemorrhoids, and so on

3.3 Mao

The time when the hand yang ming large intestine passes through the open hole is 5:00 a.m. to 7:00 a.m. (Mao). In Mao, the large intestine is prosperous. The large intestine passes and smashes through the sputum. The detoxification slag is released.

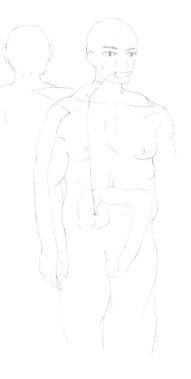

"The lungs and the large intestine are co-related." The lungs fill the whole body with full, fresh blood and then promote the large intestine into an excited state. It completes the process of absorbing the water and nutrients from the food and then discharges the dregs. It is best to have a bowel movement after getting up in the morning.

Deficiency Syndrome

Abdominal belly pain, abdominal diarrhea, weakened function of the large intestine, stiff shoulders, dull skin, sore shoulders, dry throat, wheezing, and putrefaction

Empirical Syndrome

Bloating, constipation, susceptibility to hemorrhoids, shoulder and back discomfort or pain, toothache, abnormal skin, and abnormal upper jaw

3.4 Chen

The time of foot yang ming stomach is 7:00 a.m. to 9:00 a.m. (Chen). In Chen, the stomach is prosperous. Eat breakfast at Chen. The nutrients promote a healthy body. At 7:00 to 9:00 a.m., most people have already gotten up. If you have a stomachache, stomach acid, and other problems, it is recommended that you bring nutrients to your stomach during this period because this is the time for the stomach to function. Breakfast can be porridge. A meal should be light or full.

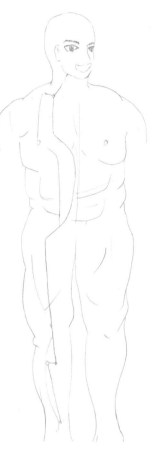

Deficiency Syndrome

Indigestion, bloating and loss of appetite, facial edema, susceptibility to hiccups, stomach pain after meals, diarrhea, or vomiting

Empirical Syndrome

Easily hungry, weak stomach, abnormal joints, abnormal appetite, dry mouth, and recurring constipation

3.5 Si

The time for foot taiyin (spleen) is 9:00 a.m. to 11:00 a.m. (Si). In Si, the spleen is prosperous and has a hematopoietic body state. "The spleen is the function of transformation and transportation; the spleen is responsible for controlling blood." The spleen is transforming among digestion, absorption, and excretion. It leads the human blood flow. "The spleen is open to the mouth; its essential is in the lips." The spleen is in good condition. Digestion and absorption occur well, and blood quality is high, so the lips are rosy. White lip marks present as the lack of blood. Dark or purple lips mean the cold pathogen into the spleen.

Deficiency Syndrome

Endocrine disorders or insufficient secretion, weakened stomach, abnormal knees, frequent insomnia, fatigue, loss of appetite, abnormal stool, abdominal distension, and so on

Empirical Syndrome

Spleen and stomach not communicating, problems in digestion and absorption, susceptibility to bloating, hiccups, headaches, fatigue, knee joint abnormalities, abnormal bowel movements, and so forth

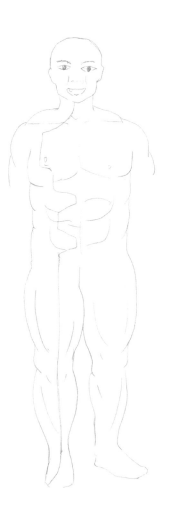

3.6 Wu

The time for Shaoyin (heart meridian of hand) is 11:00 a.m. to 1:00 p.m. (Wu). In Wu, the heart is prosperous. To soothe the spirits, you should take a short nap during Wu. "The heart is the god. It opens into the tongue; brilliance manifests in the face." The heart pushes the blood to flow and nourishes the spirit (the qi) and the sinews. It is better to sleep for a while after lunch, but there are a variety of reasons to restrain this desire.

If the conditions are allowed, just take a little nap for ten minutes. That will be helpful to your heart. Do not worry about getting fat, because that is just a short nap. It can also help gastrointestinal motility reduce any burden. Lunch should be delicious, but it should not be delicacies. The food should be warm and not raw. Neither should it be hard to bite. The meal should be 80 percent satisfaction. After lunch, drink tea to gargle. Wash off greasy hands, and then take a lunch break.

Deficiency Syndrome

Chest tightness, red face, heavy limbs, easy fatigue, poor blood circulation, chest pain, heart pain, language barriers, and so on

Empirical Syndrome

Difficulty breathing, headaches caused by poor blood circulation, dry mouth and bitterness, and palm fever

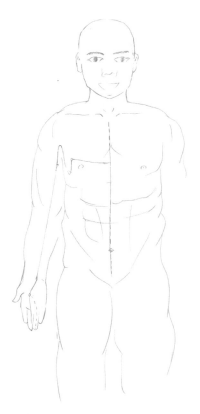

3.7 Wei

The time of small intestine meridian of hand tai yang is 1:00 to 3:00 p.m. (Wei). In Wei, the small intestine is prosperous. It is time to classify pure or turbid. Drinking water can reduce fire. The small intestine is classifying pure or turbid. The liquid is returned to the bladder. The dregs are sent to the large intestine, and the essence is transferred to the spleen. The small intestine adjusts the nutrition of the person's day in Wei time. If the small intestine is in heat, people will cough, exhaust, and fart. Drinking more water or tea at Wei is beneficial to the small intestines.

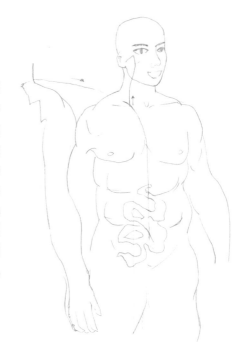

3.8 Shen

The time of the bladder meridian of foottai yang is 3:00 to 5:00 p.m. (Shen). The bladder is prosperous. In Shen, it abandons fluid in the feet, nourishing yin to comfort the body. The bladder stores water and body fluid. The water is discharged from the body, and the body fluid circulates in the body. If the bladder is in heat, it can cause bladder cough and cough to enuresis.

In Shen, the body temperature is higher. Most prominently, that happens to the person with yin deficiency. At this time, the appropriate activities help the body fluid's circulation, and drinking tea can improve nutrition in yin and release body heat. That is most effective for people with yin deficiency.

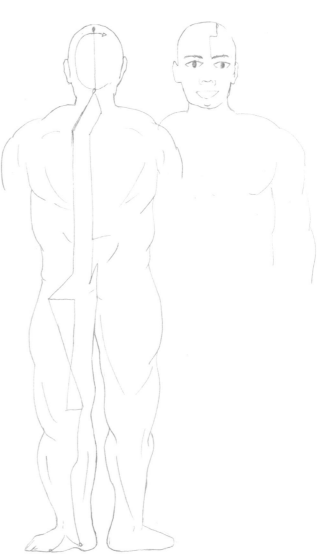

Deficiency Syndrome
Nostalgia paresthetica, low back pain, abnormal foot nerves, leg acid, acne, and frequent urination

Empirical Syndrome
Back and neck pain, sciatica, low back pain, headache, tearing, nose bleeds, and so on

3.9 You

The time for shaoyin kidney meridian of foot is 5:00 to 7:00 p.m. (You). The kidney is prosperous. In You, the kidneys are storing the essence, absorbing distillation and primordial clarification. "The kidney is the essence of the reproduction organs and the five internal organs. The kidney is the root of the innate."

The human body detoxifies during You, and the kidney enters the stage of storage essence when it is You time. At this period, it is not suitable for heavy amounts of exercise and is not suitable for drinking plenty of water.

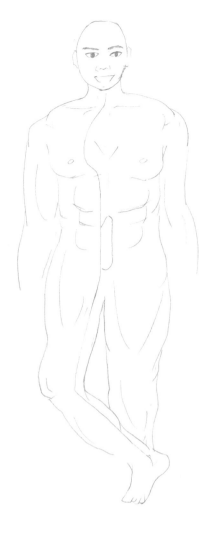

Deficiency Syndrome
Tinnitus, forgetfulness, frequent urination, acidosis of the legs, loss of libido, constipation, lack of vitality, fatigue, osteoporosis, cold hands and feet, athlete's foot, and so on

Empirical Syndrome
Tinnitus, irregular menstruation, dry mouth, abnormal blood pressure, low urine volume, dark color, turbidity, loss of libido, neurasthenia, foot sweating, genital lesions, and so on

3.10 Xu

The time of pericardium meridian is 7:00 to 9:00 p.m. (Xu). The heat is prosperous. In Xu, it is time to protect your heart and relieve your stress for smoothening your heart. "The pericardium is the outer membrane of the heart with the veins, the channel of blood flow. The pathogen cannot accommodate; otherwise the heart gets hurt."

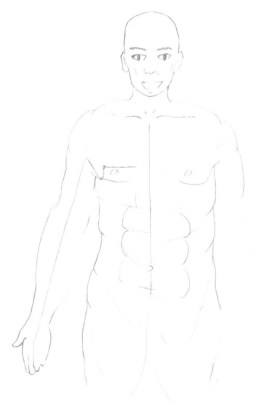

The pericardium is the protective organization of the heart but also the channel of blood. The pericardium is in the most prosperous during Xu. It can clear the pathogens around the heart and keep the heart in good condition. Be sure to keep good mood at this period: read a book, listen to music, do a spa, dance, exercise, or do tai chi. Relax and release stress.

Deficiency Syndrome

Insufficient secretion of lubricating fluid, abnormal heartbeat, asthma, insomnia along with dreams, heart disorder, speech difficulties, palm fever, and so on

Empirical Syndrome

Pericardial inflammation, chest tightness, heartache, abnormal upper jaw, lethargy, cardiovascular disease, dizziness, headache, and so on

3.11 Hai

The time for the triple-warmer meridian of hand shao yang is 9:00 to 11:00 p.m. (Hai). Triple-energizer is prosperous. When you are at the time of Hai, your veins are flowing well, and they nourish your body and beautify your outlook.

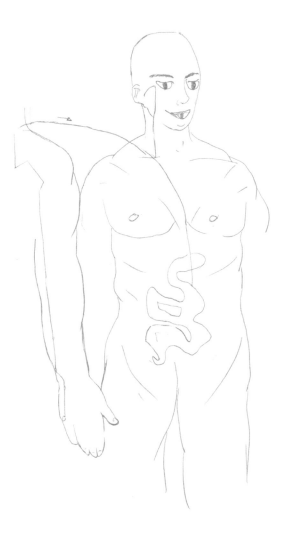

Triple-energizer is the largest entrails among the six viscera. It has the function of presiding over the qi and dredging the waterway. At the time of Hai, the triple-energizer can pass through hundreds of veins. If a person sleeps at the time of Hai, all his veins can fully rest and be nourished. That is very beneficial to the body. One-hundred-year-old people have a common feature. They all sleep at the time of Hai. If modern people don't want to sleep at this time, they can listen to music, read books, watch TV, and practice yoga, but it is best not to sleep beyond this time.

Deficiency Syndrome

Decreased immunity, fatigue, upper limb weakness, abdominal blockage, darkening of body hair, difficulty breathing, stomach cold, and so on

Empirical Syndrome

Lymphatic inflammation, migraine, shoulder aches, neck pain, fever, tinnitus, and abnormal urine

3.12 Zi

The time of shaoyang gallbladder meridian is 11:00 p.m. to 1:00 a.m. (Zi). The gallbladder is prosperous. When sleeping well during Zi time, dark circles around the eyes are not exposed.

The theory of traditional Chinese medicine believes that "the rest of the liver energy vents to the gallbladder, gathering into essence." When people sleep before the time of Zi, the gallbladder can complete the metabolism. "How clear the bile is, how clear the brain is."

When falling asleep at the time of Zi, the mind is clear, the outlook is ruddy, and there are no dark circles around the eyes. On the other hand, if you are unable to fall asleep during the time of Zi, the outlook is pale and there are black circles. Also, because of inferior metabolism of bile detoxification, it is easier to form crystals and stones.

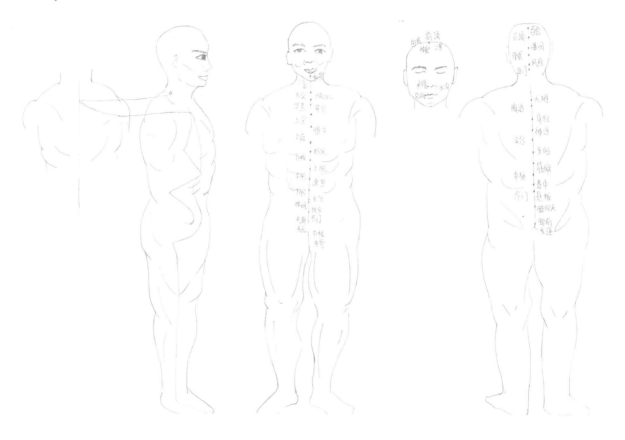

4 Organ Physiological Function and Pathological Changes

Let's talk about the physiological functions and pathological changes of the organs. Chinese medicine classifies the human viscera into five elements (wood, fire, soil, metal, and water), and they correspond to liver, heart, spleen, lung, and kidney.

4.1 Liver

Our Chinese medicine doctors call the liver "the general of the viscera," the master in strategy, as it holds and transforms blood. For example, liver blood dysfunction affects the normal activities of the human body and blood lesions. The liver cannot hold blood, making one's mind unhinged—for instance, many nightmares, unslept nights, sleepwalking, talking in dreams, and other involuntary thinking activities. If the liver function is insufficient, it will affect the blood quality and cause skin disease.

Insufficient Suffocation
The liver main function occurrence happens to have obstacles, resulting in poor qi. Qi stagnation will cause depression, suspiciousness, sadness, crying in sorrow, breast swelling, pain, discomfort, and the like.

Overventing
The liver qi is too irritating and does not have enough time to release, so the liver qi is reversed. The liver heat is inflammatory, and then the qi heat is reversed, causing the person to suddenly faint and lose consciousness. It will also affect the operation of blood and the metabolic transmission of body fluids, such as anger leading qi upward and blood stagnation in the chest.

If the liver blood is damaged and the tendons are displaced, there will be tendon weakness, limb numbness, and unfavorable joint flexion and extension. It also affects the wing of the stent. There are some dryness injuries, twitching of the limbs, angulation, and jaws closed tight.

The essence of the five viscera and six organs focusing on eyes is the top of essence. The liver is the most important viscera, as the vision comes because blood flows to eyes. If the blood is not enough, the eyes are dry, vision is unclear, and even night blindness occurs. If the liver is heat, the eye is reddish and itchy. If the liver is on fire, inflammation causes the eye's red shadows. If the liver is hepatic, wind internal movement causes the eye to be oblique. And anger is angry, qi reversal, and even vomiting of blood. The right liver suffers the wind and heat as well as kidney deficiency, and then it will tear in the wind. The liver blood deficiency or liver and kidney lack of yin will cause eyes to dry, and tears cannot flow.

4.2 Heart

The most important organ, the monarch of organs, is the foundation of life. It is the lord of the five viscera, the lord's blood, the lord's sanity. If sanity fulfills, he will tease, and if sanity is not enough, he will be sorrow. Sweat is the liquid of the heart. The body fluid is scattered in the skin and excreted by Xuanfu and sweat keratosis.

The heart of the lord of blood is nutrient of qi. The blood and the body fluid are from the same source. Therefore, the blood and sweat are homologous. If the heart is weak, then spontaneous perspiration with asthenia qi occurs, and if the heart is asthenia in yin, it then often results in sweats at night.

If the heart is asthenia qi, the face is absent pale. If the heart is asthenia blood, the face will be pale and not bright. If having blocking in heart, the face and lips will be blue and purple.

The tongue is the signal orifice of the heart. If the heart is short of yang qi, the tongue is pale and tender. If the heart is short of yin blood, the tongue is thin and tinny. If the body flames up along with inflammation, the following will happen:

- The tongue is red.
- The tongue and aphthae are sores.
- The blood has stasis.
- The tongue is purple or has freckles.
- The mental is devitalized.
- The tongue is cured or stiff.
- The aphasia is difficult.
- Recognition of words is difficult.

All kinds of dreams are related to the heart. The heart also controls speech, and in all the pathogens, the "heat pathogen" to the heart and the pericardium is the deadliest for health.

There is also a pericardium in Chinese medicine; it is also called the cardiac vesicle. It is encapsulated to protect the heart. Its function is the protection of the heart. It can prevent pathogens from entering the heart. It is the officer of joyfulness and co-related with triple-energizer. The pericardium suffers from pathogens and unusually affects the function of the heart, such as the inner flame of warmth. The symptoms are dizziness and other symptoms of devitalization. That is the heat into the pericardium.

4.3 Spleen

"The janitor of Cangjie," the spleen is responsible for transport, blood, ascendant, and purification. Secreted into the mind is called thought. Into the mouth is saliva into the four limbs of the muscles.

Responsible for Transportation
Transmit indicates transportation. Digestion indicates digestion and absorption. The spleen's major responsibility is to transport and transform the purified nutrients and water dampness, two aspects. If the spleen loses health, this will cause anorexia, abdominal distension, loose stools, burnout, edema, and sipping.

Responsible for Ascending Purification
The spleen qi ascending comes along with a healthy body. Ascending purification is a feature of spleen function. Spleen-ascending purification can also prevent visceral drooping and qi sag. If the spleen qi is not rising, it will cause dizziness, prolonged sputum, or visceral drooping.

Control Circulating Blood
If the control blood function is failure, that will cause blood in the stool, uterine bleeding, and skin purpura.

Governing Flesh
The spleen is the most important organ that determines the strength of muscles. If it is dysfunctional, the muscles are weakened, and the limbs will be tired. If there is dysfunction of spleen in transportation, then there will be a flat feeling in the mouth. If the spleen and stomach are not regulated, then there will be sweetness in the mouth.

The spleen also has the function of thinking. If the thoughts are too much, then it will cause qi stagnation and loss of appetite and function of liquid flow. If the liquid is clearer, it is called saliva. If the spleen is devitalized, then liquid consciously flows out.

4.4 Lung

"The officer as prime minister," the lung governs qi and performs respiration, governing disseminating, cleansing, and descending. The lung connects all vessels and governs management and regulation of waterways. The essence of spleen is transferred to the lungs and then spread to the skin and hair of the whole body.

The body fluid, grain, and water are infused with the inhaled qi, and the spleen scatters them down.

The lungs are on the top, so the lung's qi descending means smoothness. If the lung's qi does not descend, then there is evidence of cough, asthma, and lung's qi upward. The lungs have the function of dredging and regulating the running of the water and the road of excretion. If the lung dredging is dysfunctional, it causes edema, dysuria, oliguria, and phlegm. The lungs face all blood vessels, and it also is a heat assistant that promotes sweat regulation and blood operation. It regulates the function of transporting, running, and excreting the fluid. If in disorder, that will cause diseases of heart and lung operation, as well as excretion function. When the lungs have lesions, common symptoms are hoarseness, rheumatic arthralgia, and other throat syndromes.

4.5 Kidney

As "the officer with great power," the kidney stores essence of viscera, governs water, and controls and promotes inspiration. It is responsible for growth and development of reproduction. The kidney is water of viscera; the waist is the house of the kidney. It is the innate foundation, the viscera's and organs' foundation of the yin and yang, the residence of water and fire, and the essence storage of viscera. Kidney congenital essence is responsible for growth, development, and reproduction. It governs water, controls and promotes inspiration, governs bone, engenders marrow, and activates the brain and the body in the bone. The brilliance manifests in the hair. It frightens, impairing the kidney, amazed at the front and back of the ear. It responds for two excretions and manifests the liquid as saliva.

The essence of the kidney includes the kidney essential qi and the kidney sperm, and the kidney yin is the foundation of the human body yin. It plays a role in moisturizing and nourishing the various organs, and the kidney yang is the foundation of the human body of yang. To viscera and organs, it plays a role in energized catalyst effect. Kidney yin and yang are mutually dependent on each other and maintains the physiological balance of the human body.

Kidney yin and yang are the foundation of yin and yang of various organs. If the kidney yin and yang imbalance will affect the balance of yin and yang of organs, other viscera's yin and yang disorders will affect the yin and yang of the kidney. This kind of disease is called "long illness effects kidney."

The opening and closing of the bladder are also controlled by the kidney yin and yang. If there is dysfunction of closing, it will cause edema, dysuria, or increased urine output. When the orifice is opened in the ear and two yins, the emotion is fear. In the liquid is saliva. The ear can hear. That relies on the essence of the kidney to support, so the kidney opens into ears.

The two yin of the ears refers to the vagina, genitals, and anus. All are affected by the qi transformation of the kidney to play a role. All are afraid of being frightened, fear of qi descending, and shock by qi chaos. Kidney deficiency causes throat dryness.

Chinese medicine believes that if the gallbladder, small and large intestine, stomach, bladder, and triple-energizer do not operate normally, it will cause the following diseases:

- The gallbladder is "the official of Zhongzheng." Anger, frustration, and resentment causes gallbladder disease.
- The small intestine is "the official of Sheng." Small intestine disease can cause sadness, destroy goods, and control others.
- The stomach is "the official of Cangjie." Stomach diseases can easily cause anger, worry, and overthinking.
- The large intestine is "the official of conduction." Abnormal operation of the large intestine will cause sadness and worry.
- The bladder is "the official of the state." The diseases are anxiety and unsecured. Children will be afraid; adults will be suspicious and jealous.

4.6 Triple-Energizer

Triple-energizer is "the official of the decision." It is the regulating body's vital energy and water-liquid passageway. It spreads the water to the whole body through the lung and heart cardiopulmonary action, warming the muscles, sinews, and bones. It includes the spleen and stomach as well as decomposition of grain and water and discharge of blood.

It also includes the liver, gallbladder and kidney, large and small intestine, bladder, and genitals. It is responsible for separating the clarity from the turbidity, secreting turbidity, and excreting water and dregs. If the above functions do not work properly, the body will develop various diseases. The incidence of each person is different.

Chinese medicine believes that the main causes of illness are roughly three aspects.

External causes are wind, cold, heat, humidity, dryness, and fire. They are related to the climate. Internal causes are joy, anger, anxiety, worry, grief, fear, and fright. They are related to psychological factors. Neither internal nor external causes overeating, excessive sexual intercourse, and excessive fatigue.

Based on our long-term experience, let's look at what Parkinson's has to do with the seven emotions. The relationship between the seven emotions and the visceral qi and blood, along with different emotional moods, have different effects on the internal organs. And the changes in the viscera in qi and blood also affect the emotions. For example, the emotion in the heart is the joy, the emotion in the liver is the anger, and the concentration in the spleen is the thought. The emotion in the kidney is the fear, but if the blood is overrun, it becomes anger. If it is insufficient, blood becomes fearful. If the liver qi is deficiency, it will be fearful. If asthenia is hepatic qi, it will be anger. If deficiency of cardiac qi, it will be sad, but if asthenia of cardiac qi, it will be unstoppable laughter. The seven emotions are closely related to the viscera and blood.

Characteristics to Cure the Seven Emotions
Direct injury in the internal organs affects viscera qi movement. Overwhelming joy impairs the heart. Overjoying will make the mind scatter. With inability to focus, there is sadness and anger.

Rage impairs the liver. Excessive anger will make liver qi flow upward. The asthenia of liver yang or the inflammation of the liver will damage the blood of the liver. Anxiety impairs the spleen. Excessive anxiety will affect the spleen, causing it to lose functionalities, like stagnation of qi, learning, concentration, and memorization.

Sadness impairs the lungs. Excessive sorrow wounds the lungs and causes sadness. Fear impairs the kidneys. Excessive fear will wound the kidneys, lose the kidney's qi, and cause anxiety and feelings of being threatened.

According to the experience we have explored in the course of treatment in Parkinson's for more than a decade, the disease has a deep relationship with the seven emotions of the human body, causing the body not to or lessen producing dopamine. Therefore, there is no way to transmit information through the cells into the brain. It produces the symptoms of Parkinson's as following.

In this world, everything could be happening with a new beginning. The wisdom of Chinese medicine for five thousand years has made us have a superior experience in treatment. With the ancient wisdom, ancestral acupuncture with kung fu manipulating acupoints can solve the following symptoms of Parkinson, and there are no side effects during treatment so almost all patients can rehabilitate or relieve symptoms. Because these physical dysfunctions on the five viscera and six organs, the consequence is unable to perform at work. Parkinson's is one of the affected diseases.

The most incomprehensible solution for Western medicine is how to loosen muscles that are tightened tightly as well as eliminate the tremors and transfer the function of dopamine.

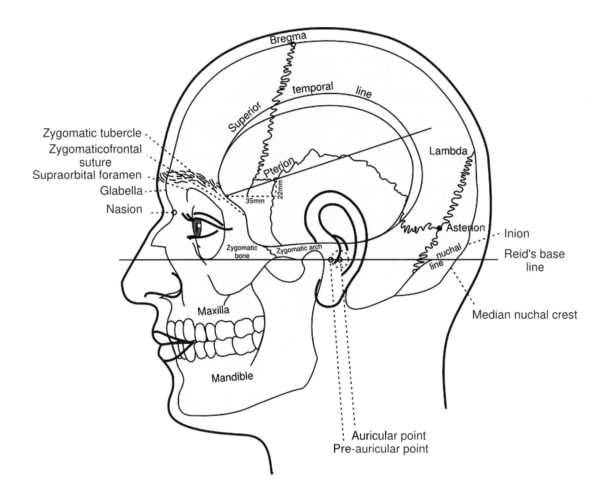

Because the patient is not the only the problem that the midbrain cells can't pass to the brain, it also is just as implied that Parkinson's comprehensive causes five viscera and six organs to produce systemic lesions.

4.7 Characteristics of Parkinson's Disease

Whole-body muscle cramps (from head to toe) make the person's shape look like a bent waist, like severely holding a cane. With their vision, they can only see their own toes, causing all kinds of internal organs of the body to produce various symptoms as described above about the liver, heart, spleen, lungs, and kidneys. It causes various organ diseases as described above because they are not functioning properly.

Some people are prone to fall and experience body pain because of the muscles tightening. There is a static hand trembling. (Not everyone is the same; some people are not shaking.) Breaking the steps is another symptom. One step is for normal people. Parkinson's patients take four or five steps.

The face will be stiff and expressionless. The tongue is stiff, and the speech is unclear. Every muscle in the body is stiff and minutely painful. There is difficulty in swallowing. The person feels desperate and lethargic.

Under current Western medical law, the Western medical treatment on the market mainly has patients take dopamine, even though they only take a onetime check and then implant the antishake microchip into the body. They can't fundamentally solve all the problems to make Parkinson's patients recover.

In fact, Parkinson's patients are far more than these nine syndromes. Many patients potentially have countless diseases of the above-mentioned five viscera and six organs.

5 Case of Treatment

According to the 2010 American scientific magazine, *Scientific*, in the Japanese edition in the 1980s, the United States gathered more than ten thousand scientists specializing in Parkinson's disease research. It has been nearly forty years since its inception, and many large-scale private companies have been researching ever since then. Research is continuing.

5.1 2007

After I reviewed this news, I recalled that I successfully rehabilitated a seventy-five-year-old elderly Parkinson patient in Japan at the Ginza Clinic in Tokyo in 2007. After seeing the reports in the above magazines, we returned to the elder who was treated three years ago.

Knowing him is fascinating. He is talkative. He walks like a normal person and often participates in some social entertainment and activities after retirement, such as singing karaoke, playing cards, fishing, and so forth. He often does acupoint manipulation to stay healthy. A happy life looks like a fish living in happiness. We all are very joyful with each other after three years of reunion.

At that time, we also used the mobile phone to take a video. Unfortunately, after arriving in the United States, maybe my mobile phone was too beautiful with the golden case. My phone accidentally disappeared, but there was no problem. In the future, we can record my Parkinson's treatment in America to prove our technology.

I recalled that, three years ago, his friend introduced him to me. His face was stunned. His facial muscles tightened. He could not smile. His tongue was rigid.

His speech was unclear. His muscles were tightened. His steps were broken. His appearance was miserable, and he almost lost hope in life.

At this age, he had never experienced acupuncture. In order to rule out his fear of acupuncture, we used the ancestral kung fu acupoint manipulation to treat him. He insisted on two or three hours of treatment a day.

I heard that he was already hospitalized at the most famous hospital in Japan. After our treatment, in less than a month, his condition was obviously improved. I heard that his doctor at the hospital was very confused and astonished.

5.2 2016

In addition to the Japanese example above, we have many successful examples.

For instance, in 2016, a Parkinson's patient was introduced to the Cupertino USA clinic. A seventy-two-year-old man has spent six years as a Parkinson's patient. He is a software engineer who has been well educated in the United States. He has a PhD in computer science with fifty years of professional working experience. The following is his statement:

Six years ago, a neurosurgeon diagnosed me with Parkinson's disease. After I learned more, I know that this is a degenerative disease with a no-end treatment. At my age, the only comfort is that the disease process is slow. I can live a natural life before the terrible end of Parkinson's disease.

My stuttering, unstable walking, and drooling are symptoms of Parkinson's disease. Because I can't keep my back straight, I cannot walk straight, and I have to lower my body. Why am I taking a small step? This is to keep my speed of balance, which makes me more unstable. I fall on average once a week. When I get into an unstable position, I am anxious to tell myself, "I want to stand up!" But the fall is a foregone conclusion. Obviously because I used my left knee habitually, my left knee was always in tiredness. My legs are too weak, I have difficulty getting up when I get up, and all the muscles in my head and neck are shaking.

Taking Western drugs (Levodopa, an anti-Parkinson medication) can cause drowsiness and constipation. Later I went to seek the help of Parkinson's experts to treat the disease. The same drugs are used by experts, but at higher doses. This medicine seems to have some effect, but there is no help for my drooling effect.

Recently I experienced a treatment from Chinese medicine acupuncture and came to help Americans learn the treatment of Parkinson's disease. That year, I was diagnosed with damage caused by Parkinson's disease, and my organs have been weakened. I have undergone a series of acupuncture treatments to strengthen the circulation of the system inside the body and immune system to help me recover. Through the stimulation of more than twenty therapies, the tension of my muscles is restored by relaxing the muscles.

6 Comparison of Treatment

6.1 Chinese Medicine Treatment

As far as the meridians and acupoint maps mentioned above are concerned, thousands of years ago, Chinese people used to treat diseases according to these. (In the past, we also had traditional Chinese medicine surgery. We could also operate with splints to treat fractures. On the contrary, with the most advanced Western medicine, they consider that the treatment method of plaster is not so good as the result of natural recovery of Chinese medicine splint.)

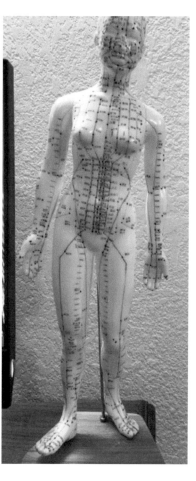

Through acupuncture and acupoint manipulation of these meridians, acupuncture points (the meridian outside the epidermis, internal viscera) stimulate the internal function of the body through the meridian. The method of restoring health to patients has prevailed around the world now. In the United States, there are dozens of Chinese medicine acupuncture universities run by Americans because acupuncture and acupressure therapy is very effective for the human body.

As we all know, the three American scientists who won the Nobel Prize in 2017 have long-term research and proved that the "Zi-Wu streamnote" described in the "HuangDi NeiJing" ("the human body clock"), the oldest medical book in China three thousand years ago, is correct. Therefore, in the famous hospitals and even the military in the United States, there are Chinese acupuncturists and acupressure manipulation to treat many diseases that are difficult for Western medicine to reach that kind of threat.

According to the process of the development of thousands of years, human beings are part of the natural world. Diseases are closely related to the changes of nature and the rhythm of life and work, so the treatment should come from the natural method to regain health. In today's modern society, people use super-high speed on work and learning. That destroys the natural regulations in the human body. Therefore, in order to restore one's health, it is necessary to return one by getting close to nature.

However, there is traditional Chinese medicine acupuncture, acupressure, cupping, scraping, moxibustion, Chinese medicine, and so on. Also the other great effective treatments seem simple. In fact, to be capable to cure diseases at any time, one must extensively learn and practice for more than ten years, so as the understanding of the society. The doctor's plenty of life experience, not just memorized acupuncture meridians and acupunctured points, is counted to be successful in this field!

6.2 Mang Zhen

The Mang Zhen is a treatment using needles of more than seventy centimeters. In my teens, under the strict training and supervision of my father, I mastered one of the ancient Chinese techniques, Mang Zhen, to puncture the Dai Mai (带脉), a channel that crosses inner organs in the abdomen from one side to reach the Dai Mai on the other side of the body. (To increase power, do a thousand push-ups per day.)

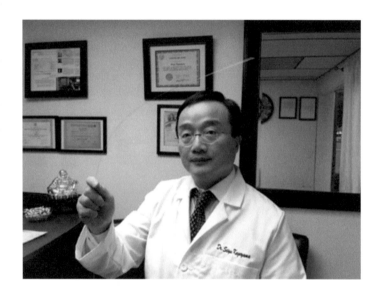

6.3 Current Western Medical Treatment

6.3.1 Gene Therapy

The general concept of gene therapy is to use a noninfectious virus (such as an adeno-associated virus) as a vector to deliver a gene fragment into a target cell. These genes can help create enzymes that improve Parkinson's disease and protect the brain from harm [59] [138].

As of 2010, there are four cases in the Parkinson's disease world widely treated with gene therapy [59], but the side effects and effects of treatment remain to be observed [59]. As of 2011, one of the experimenters indicate an improvement, but this trial drug company, Neurologix, declared bankruptcy in March 2012 [140].

6.3.2 Neuroprotective Therapy

Neuro maintenance is currently one of the most cutting-edge topics of research in Parkinson's disease, and several chemicals have been reported to have therapeutic potential [59], but no substance has officially claimed the deceleration of degeneration [59].

The substances still under research includes antiapoptotic substances (Omigapil, CEP-1347), antiglutamate drugs, monoamine oxidase inhibitors (Hilicillin, Rasagiline), mitochondrial bioenergy conversion agents (Coenzyme Q10, creatine), calcium channel blockers (Ai Lei Xiping), growth factors (GDNF), and so forth. [59]. There have also been studies of α-Synuclein vaccine PD01A, which has now entered human clinical trials [141]. Fatal side effects include psychotic drugs nausea syndrome [6], so it is no longer being used [6].

At present, some manufacturers have developed intravenous and intestinal sustained-release technologies to make L-dopa stable and release deceleration. Studies have shown that sustained release agents can effectively reduce dyskinesia compared to traditional dosage forms [6][71]. Most patients must take L-dopa for life, and they will generally experience the side effects in the motor due to this product in the future [6].

6.3.3 Dopamine Receptor Agonist

In addition to L-dopa, several dopamine receptor agonists can also bind to postsynaptic dopamine receptors and thereby achieve therapeutic effects [6]. These drugs were originally used to improve the patient from the side effects after L-dopa, but mostly now they are used for delaying the treatment of initial motor symptoms [6][72], and the use of this product at the later stage of sickness can improve the symptoms (power off state) ("off" state) [6]. Drugs for dopamine receptor agonists include bromocriptine, pergolide, pramipexole, ropinirole, cabergoline, apomorphine, and lisuride [73].

Dopamine receptor agonists may cause serious or minor side effects, including hypersomnia, hallucinations, insomnia, nausea, and constipation [6]. Some patients have side effects even at very low doses. Then doctors are advised to consider changing the medicine [6]. Dopamine receptor agonists can delay the development of motor symptoms, although the efficacy is not as strong as L-dopa [6] but sufficiently control the initial symptoms [20].

The price of such drugs is generally more expensive than L-dopa [20]. Young patients taking this class of drugs have less dyskinesia, and side effects get higher along with age [20]. This class of drugs is commonly used to treat initial symptoms to delay the use of L-dopa [20]. It produces impulsive control disorders that are stronger than L-dopa, and patients may experience morbid gluttony, sexual impulses, gambling, and shopping [40].

Apomorphine can be used to decelerate the symptoms of off power and dyskinesia in the late course of the disease [6]. The available alternation treatment method includes intermittent injection and continuous subcutaneous infusion [6]. Because side effects such as confusion and hallucinations are quite common, the treatment with apomorphine must be closely monitored [6]. Lisuride and Rotigotine are two dopamine agonists used through dermal patches that are useful not only for early patients but also for patients with severe off power [71].

6.3.4 Monoamine Oxidase Inhibitor

Monoamine oxidase inhibitors include safinamide, selegiline, and rasagiline, which increase dopamine content of basal ganglia by inhibiting monoamine oxidase B (MAO-B). A dopamine neuron-secreted MAO-B will explain dopamine, so a decrease in MAO-B activity will increase the L-dopa content of the striatum (part of the basal ganglia) [6].

Just like a dopamine receptor agonist, treating a patient with a monoamine oxidase inhibitor can improve motor syndrome and delay the need for L-dopa at early stages of patients, but it has more side effects than dopamine receptor agonists, and the effect is not as good as L-dopa. Although studies have shown that monoamine oxidase inhibitors can reduce the severity of a patient's condition between off and on states, there are not much more in advance studies of monoamine oxidase inhibitors [6]. A preliminary research indicates that the combination of Selegiline and L-dopa may lead to increased mortality but remains to be confirmed [6].

6.3.5 Nerve Transplantation

Since the early 1980s, attempts have been made to transplant fetal, porcine, carotid, or retinal tissue to the substantia nigra to repair neural connections between the substantia nigra and the brain [59]. Although there is an initial evidence that transplanted dopamine neurons to midbrain may be effective, double-blind trials currently show no long-term benefit [59]. In addition, transplanted tissue may release excess dopamine, causing dystonia [142].

Stem cell transplantation is the focus of today's research because stem cells are easy to manipulate, and experiments in monkeys have shown that animals survive successfully, also reducing behavioral abnormalities [59] [143]. However, the use of embryos is still quite controversial to date [59] and may therefore be directed toward the use of less controversial inducible pluripotent stem cells (iPS) [59].

7 The Conference of Parkinson's Disease and Treatment Evidence

After reading the 2010 issue of the *American Science Journal* and the Parkinson's report in the Japanese edition, I really wanted to share this technology around the world. So we are looking at the web for the opportunities to publish this paper at an international conference and finally on the internet. The 2010 World Symposium on Acupuncture and Moxibustion, hosted by the World Federation of Acupuncture and Moxibustion, will be held in San Francisco.

At that time, the conference had already passed the deadline of publication of the paper, but we were eager to publish the results of this treatment. After the preparatory office of the conference reviewed our papers, they determined the value of our unique content. Finally they exceptionally agreed to our participation. I highly appreciate that they gave me this opportunity.

At that time, the conference agreed to give me a fifteen-minute speech. Because the content of the speech was the first-time example of Parkinson's treatment in the world, we had an enthusiastic response at the conference. The audience and I had done a lot of academic exchanges, and the scene was very exciting.

Although I was scheduled to be the last one to speak, my speech was only fifteen minutes before lunch, but after more than thirty minutes of communication with participants, everyone was unwilling to leave in that atmosphere. In addition, in my introducing the "mountain needle," the description of the treatment of the needles of more than seventy centimeters had made the meeting a new exhilarated scene.

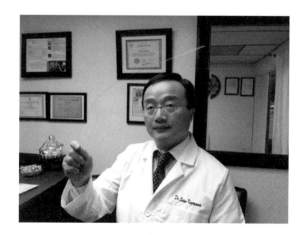

"An acupuncturist holding a long needle."

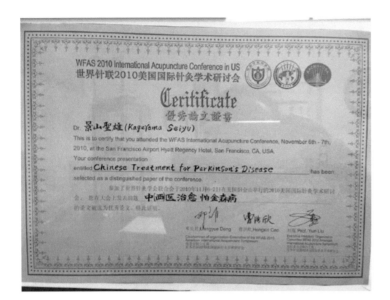

After the two-day conference, the president of the general assembly awarded the Parkinson's Therapy Excellent Paper Award. (And of course, other doctors won the Excellent Paper Award in other fields.)

After the conference, I saw lots of the talents of Chinese medicine practitioners in the United States gaining such strong momentum. Then I had the idea for further promoting Parkinson's treatment technology in the United States and decided to have prosperity develop in the United States.

Later I obtained a master's degree in Chinese medicine and a California Chinese medicine license in the United States. The news of my Parkinson's treatment was spread wide. Harvard Medical School invited me to attend a world-famous expert meeting.

While treating other diseases in the United States, we later focused on the treatment of Parkinson's and achieved a great response. In addition to treating Parkinson's patients in our own clinic, we also performed on-site treatment demonstrations at the Parkinson's patient meeting in the San Francisco community. All of those showed effective results on the spot.

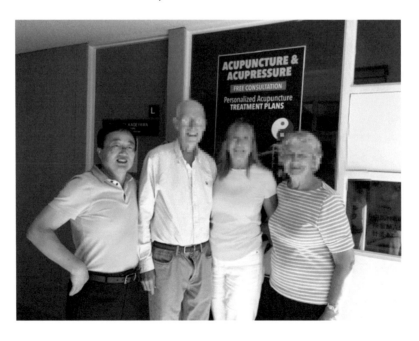

This photo was taken at the Stanford University Pediatric Hospital, next door to the Jin Clinic, after Parkinson's disease treatment.

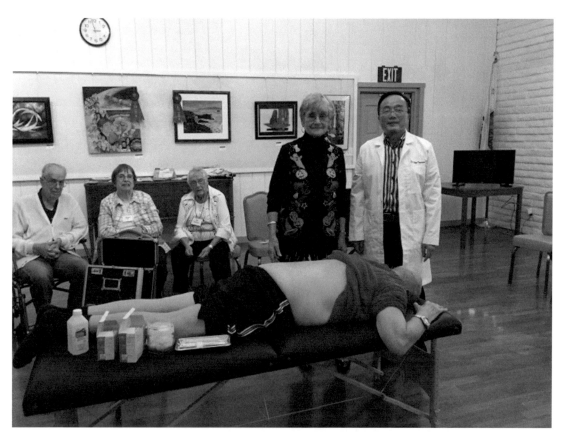

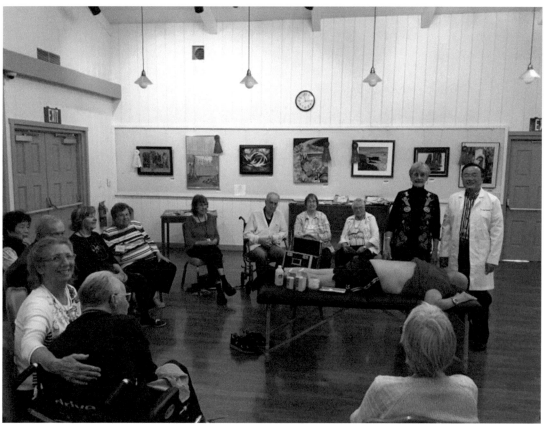

*This photo was taken at a live demonstration of treatment
at the Parkinson's Party in South Bay, San Francisco.*

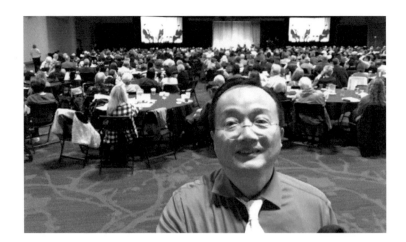

In May 2016, the author was invited to participate in the thousand-person Parkinson's Patient Conference organized by the Michael J. Fox Foundation.

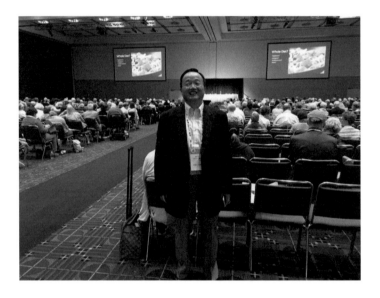

This photo was taken in 2016 at the Parkinson's Conference in Portland with five thousand attendees.

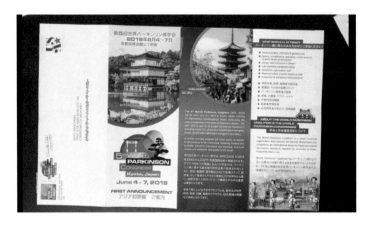

This photo shows the America's Parkinson Disease Association's invitation letter from New York to participate in the 2019 Japan Kyoto World Parkinson's Patient Conference with ten thousand attendees.

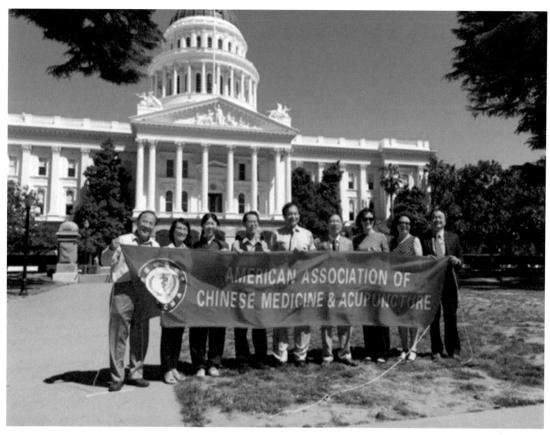

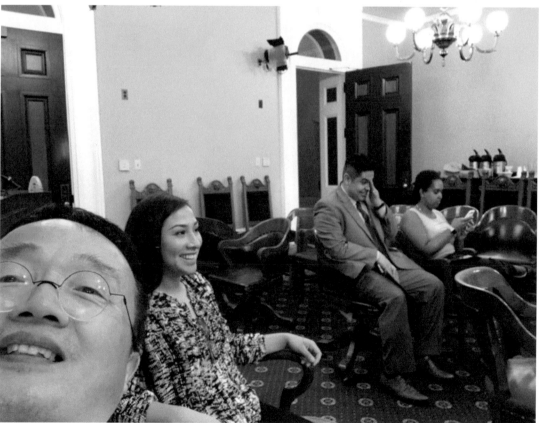

This photo shows the 2017 California state government in Sacramento promoting Chinese medicine, offering government officials a free treatment.

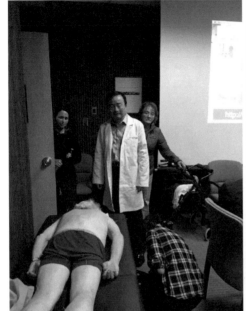
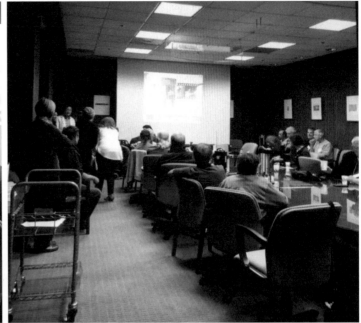
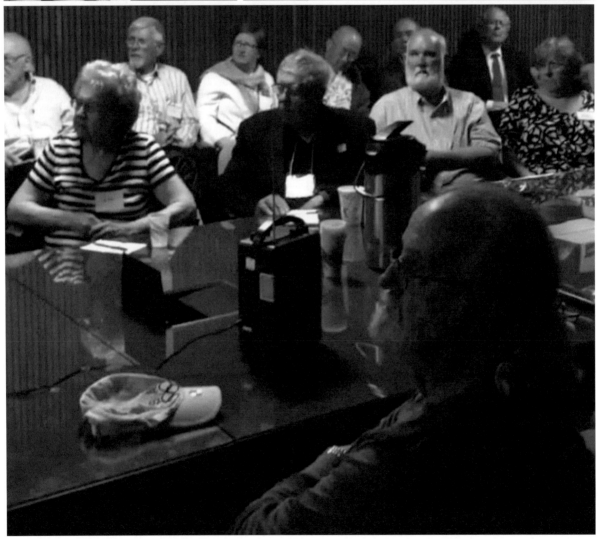

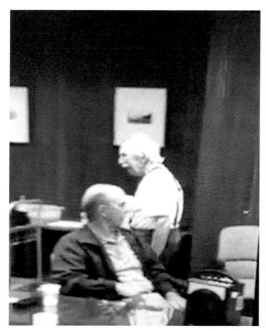

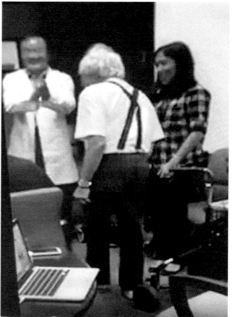

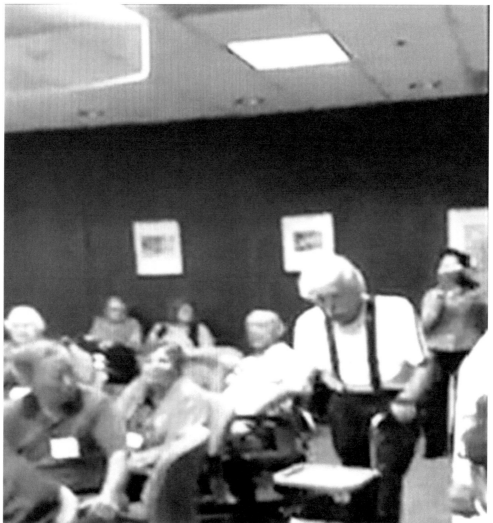

Patients and doctors are cheering and calling it a miracle.

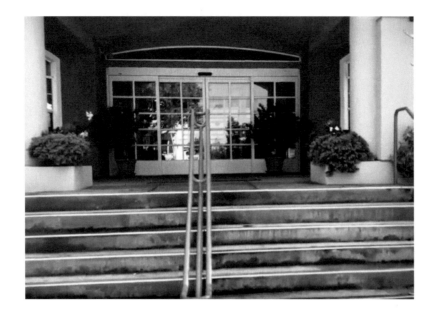

This photo shows the VA treatment center, Parkinson's branch, in San Francisco after a treatment. The patient does not need a trolley on the scene and does not fall either.

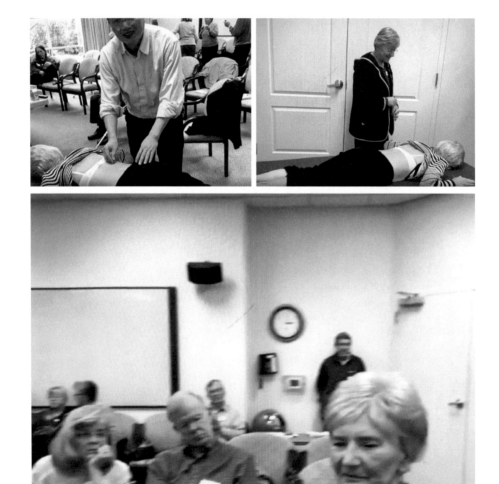

This photo shows the San Francisco Mulberry Parkinson's group live demonstration of treatment and achievements.

Summarizing the experience and great results of treating Parkinson's for more than ten years, it turns out that the ancient ancestral Chinese medicine acupuncture, moxibustion, and acupressure carried out specific syndrome differentiation and treatment. Dopamine cells can be produced by treating all the lesions produced by fourteen meridians (all organs) one by one. Parkinson's patients should be able to be fully restored to health.

8 References

Parkinson's Disease. Information Page. NINDS. 2016-06-30 [2016-07-18].

Sveinbjornsdottir, S. "The Clinical Symptoms of Parkinson's Disease." *Journal of Neurochemistry* (July 11, 2016). doi:1111/jnc.13691.PMID 27401947.

Jones, H. Royden. *The Netter Collection of Medical Illustrations: A Compilation of Paintings.* 2nd ed. Philadelphia: Saunders Elsevier, 2013.

Kalia, L. V., and A. E. Lang. "Parkinson's Disease." *Lancet* 386, no. 9996 (August 8, 2015): 896–982. Doi:10.1016/s0140-6736 (14)61393-3. PMID 25904081..

Barranco Quintana, J. L., M. F. Allam, A. S. Del Castillo, and R. F. Navajas. "Parkinson's Disease and Tea: A Quantitative Review." *Journal of the American College of Nutrition* 28, no. 1 (February 2009): 1–6. doi:10.1808/07315724.2009.1071 9754. PMID 19571153.

The National Collaborating Centre for Chronic Conditions (编). *Symptomatic Pharmacological Therapy in Parkinson's Disease.* London: Royal College of Physicians, 2006.

Barichella M., E. Cereda, and G. Pezzoli. "Major Nutritional Issues in the Management of Parkinson's Disease." *Mov. Disord.* 24, no. 13 (October 2009): 1881–92. doi:10.1002/mds.22705. PMID 19691125.

Ahlskog, J. E. "Does Vigorous Exercise Have a Neuroprotective Effect in Parkinson Disease?" *Neurology* 77, no. 3 (July 19, 2011): 288–94. doi:10.121/wnl. 0b013e8225ab66. PMC 3136051. PMID 21768599.

GBD 2013 Mortality and Causes of Death, Collaborators. "Global, Regional, and National Age–Sex Specific All Cause and Cause-Specific Mortality for 240 of Death, 1990–2013: A Systematic Analysis for the Global Burden of Disease Study 2013." *Lancet* 385 (December 17, 2014): 117–71. doi:10.1016/ S0140-6736(14)61682-2. PMC 4340604.

9 Supplementary Data

Appreciation Letter from Lymphoma Disease Patient

April 23, 2014

To whom it may concern,

I am a longtime non-Hodgkin's lymphoma patient who has had success with acupuncture treatment. I have had non-Hodgkin's lymphoma (indolent B-cell lymphoma) since November 2004. During the first years, my tumors increased, although not to the point of required treatment. I started acupuncture treatment in October 2008. In 2011, I had several CT scans to determine further growth of the cancer. At that point, my oncologist said that tumor growth over the past two years had been minimal. In 2013, I had another CT scan that showed the same result: no growth or increase in cancer cells. I attribute this to acupuncture treatment.

I have been treated several times by Mr. Kageyama Jing. I found him to be an excellent and highly skilled acupuncturist, and I recommend him highly.

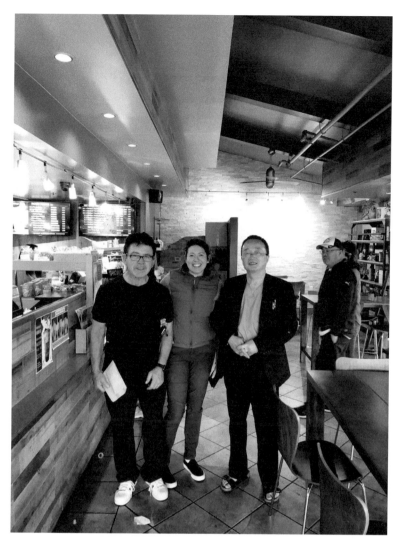

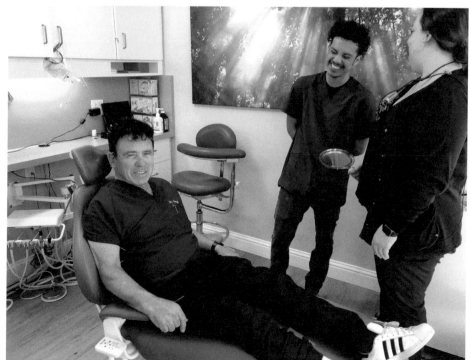

Dear Mr. Kageyama,

I can't express my gratitude for your help in improving my movement disorder due to my Parkinson's disease. With your skills in accupuncture I have been able to reduce my medication by a fourth of the amount I was taking. In addition, your dedication to my health has surpassed the commitment of any doctor that I have worked with in the past. The accupuncture treatment I received from you has returned the quality of life back to me. You have beautifully blended eastern and western medicine, so they can compliment each other.

Thank you,

Dr. Frank Grimaldi

For many years I struggled with the symptoms of Parkinson's. Western doctors could only diagnose me and chart the progression of the disease. It was very disappointing. As a result, I sought out Chinese medicine practitioners and tried a few acupuncturists. The results varied and often times I felt I was not getting the results I needed. Then I read about Mr. S Kageyama and was so impressed by the work that he had done as a specialist in treating Parkinson's that I decided to fly to California and undergo an intensive treatment program with him. For the first time, I found practitioner who treated my entire body and mind through ancient methods as well as modern scientific theory. Mr. S Kageyama is both skilled in his practice and demonstrates the highest level of personal care toward his patients. After the first few treatments I began to feel Improvement in my condition and my overall flexibility and ability to move. Mr. S Kageyama also taught me about the root causes of my condition and the need to change my lifestyle and showed me ways to reduce tension and stress. The most important thing I have received since starting to be treated by Mr. S Kageyama is a greater sense of hope. I now see that there is a pathway toward Improvement of my condition and look forward to further progress. Thank you, Mr. S Kageyama.

-Anonymous